T5-DIG-966

WINNING
THE COLD WAR

ANNE HUNT

Edited by Eric Mein, M.D.

A Note to the Reader

The information in this book is not presented as prescription for the treatment of disease. Application of the medical information found in the Cayce readings and interpreted herein should be undertaken only under the supervision of a physician.

Other Books in This Series

WEIGHT NO MORE: A Weight-Loss Program That Can Work
SAVING YOUR SKIN: Secrets of Healthy Skin and Hair

Copyright © 1990
by the
Edgar Cayce Foundation.
All rights reserved.
ISBN 0-87604-261-2

First Printing: October, 1990
Printed in the U.S.A.

Table of Contents

Preface by Mark Thurston, Ph.D.   V

Introduction by Eric Mein, M.D.   IX

Chapter One   Our Bodies Know Best   1

Chapter Two   Common Cold or Flu?   4

Chapter Three   Prevention Is Possible   9

Chapter Four   The Three R's of Cure   31

Chapter Five   Remedies for Relief   41

Chapter Six   Winning the Seven-Day
                   Cold War   50

Conclusion   53

Appendix A   Who Was Edgar Cayce?   55

Appendix B   How the A.R.E. Can Help
                   You   57

Appendix C   Where to Find the Remedies
                   and Ingredients   59

Appendix D   Edgar Cayce Reading on the
                   Common Cold   60

Know that there is within yourself all healing that may be
accomplished for your body . . .   **Based on reading 4021-1**

EDGAR CAYCE
PIONEER IN HOLISTIC HEALTH CARE

PREFACE

It's no secret that our society is in the midst of a health care crisis. The problem is partly economic, as we struggle to find ways to pay for the high level of care made possible by medical technology. It's also a research crisis, as scientists look for cures to new diseases such as AIDS. Those are the sorts of problems that make the headlines. Those are the challenges that are clearly evident.

But our health care crisis has more subtle features, too—aspects that are easy to miss but just as important. For example, how much guarantee can doctors give us for our health? How much responsibility are we willing to accept *for ourselves?* Are there some ailments for which *self-care* is not only more economical but also more likely to produce the results we want?

Another elusive feature of our society's health care crisis is in our attitude toward health and healing itself. Recent decades have seen an explosion of alternative health services, many of them claiming to follow a more natural or a more holistic approach. The success of some of these new methods makes us wonder about the validity of the familiar medical model. Is the body really more or less a machine that gets fixed like a balky appliance or a malfunctioning vehicle? Or is the human being a rich, complex mixture of body, mind, and spirit where problems at one level must be addressed at all three?

Working in the first four-and-a-half decades of the twentieth century, Edgar Cayce was a tremendous resource that we can now draw upon to meet the modern crisis in health care. His approach and methods for health maintenance and healing feature self-care that is often, yet not always, in conjunction with a physician's guidance. He was truly a pioneer of the contemporary holistic health movement and ahead of his times in pointing out the attitudinal, emotional, and spiritual components of disease.

Although best known as a "psychic" (or "the sleeping prophet," referring to his occasional predictions about world conditions), Cayce might be better labeled as a "clairvoyant diagnostician" or an "intuitive physician." The point with these descriptive terms is to emphasize first that Cayce's work was principally diagnostic and prescriptive. He was not a healer nor did he have office hours to see patients the way a doctor would. The cases that he took, the people who came to him for help were almost invariably those who had unsuccessfully tried the traditional medical approaches of their day and came to Cayce as a last resort, asking, "What's *really* wrong with me? What treatments—no matter how unusual—will bring relief and healing?"

But as the descriptive labels for Cayce also emphasize, his method of meeting those requests was intuitive. He had no formal medical school training. Yet he was apparently able to alter his consciousness in such a way that he could see clairvoyantly the real origins of afflictions (physical, mental, and spiritual). What's more, he could then prescribe natural and holistic treatment procedures—sometimes requiring the involvement of a physician or other health care professional, but often needing only a self-care regimen.

The material came through as lengthy discourses (called "readings"), which were stenographically recorded and then transcribed. Most of the information was given for specific individuals and their afflictions, but on occasion there were readings given on particular health topics which contained universally applicable information.

This book is one of a series of volumes in which common ailments and health difficulties are examined. Each topic addresses information given by Cayce which is principally focused upon self-care. The author, Anne Hunt, has carefully researched those readings on the respective health concern, focusing on the treatment procedures that were suggested to many different people as well as those recommendations that were clearly indicated for general use. Her research compilation and writing go a long way toward making these helpful methods accessible to us all. You'll find all the books in this series highly readable and very practical.

Anne's collaborator is Dr. Eric Mein, who served as medical editor. Sometimes Cayce's language requires the insight of a trained physician to translate concepts into modern terminology. Often there are new findings in medical research that shed light on one of Cayce's ideas. Eric has skillfully added that dimension to the creation of this book.

This particular volume in the series focuses on one of the most universal ailments—the common cold—along with an even more debilitating malady, the flu. The Cayce readings don't claim to have an absolute cure for either of these viral infections, but they do offer a highly practical, self-care approach to prevention as well as treatment.

Mark Thurston, Ph.D.
Association for Research and Enlightenment, Inc.

INTRODUCTION

No one is a stranger to the common cold and to all its attendant symptoms and miseries. Upper respiratory infections, along with influenza, account for almost half of all acute illness in this country—occurring more frequently than headaches, dental conditions, digestive disturbances, backaches, rashes, sprains, and contusions combined.

Despite the fact that only 5-15% of these colds are ever brought to the attention of a health practitioner, Americans spend more than one billion dollars annually on the more than 800 over-the-counter oral cold medications now offered, as well as scores of sprays, lozenges, and elixirs found on drugstore shelves. Given the importance of self-care in treating the common cold, many individuals have wished there was a better understanding of this process and a more natural approach to home treatment.

The holistic approach to the common cold and flu that you'll find within these pages comes from a unique source—the readings of Edgar Cayce, one of the foremost psychics of the twentieth century. The majority of his readings dealt with the physical concerns of individuals who sought his advice.

From among the health topics he addressed, the common cold holds a unique position. In addition to hundreds of references to the common cold in the information given for those seeking relief, it was one of the few ailments covered by a general reading on the condition itself (see Appendix D).

Calling the cold "one of the most erratic conditions that may be considered as an ill to the human body" (902-1),[1] the readings acknowledge that the cold is caused by a contagious germ. We now know that over 200 different viruses from six virus families account for the majority of these infections. The illnesses that they produce range from a few sniffles to potentially life-threatening strains of influenza.

Often, when the cause of our illness clearly has such an external source, we feel that there is not much we can do either to prevent it or to work to hasten the end of our symptoms. The readings, however, invite us to reconsider Pasteur's remark, "The germ is nothing, the soil everything." Reflecting on this concept, we are advised to stop "trying to remove blades of grass and not removing that that grows same—for, with the fertile soil,

---

[1] The Edgar Cayce readings have each been assigned a two-part number for identification. The first digits indicate the specific number assigned to the topic or individual obtaining the reading. Since many received more than one reading, the second set of digits following the hypen indicates the number in that particular series of readings.

same continues to put forth those hindrances as here." (137-95) This admonition from the readings makes a clear statement. Don't just treat the symptoms—correct the causes.

While these readings have good ideas to help with symptom relief, they go even further in suggesting ways to help restore balance to the body more quickly. These tools work with patterns of circulation and elimination, the immune system, our acid/alkaline balance, and attitude. Since advice for the prevention of both colds and flu overlapped, both sicknesses are combined together in this booklet.

These same concepts can be invaluable to us even when we are healthy, as they form the cornerstone of the optimal approach to working with any ailment: *prevention.*

What kinds of unique perspectives did the readings offer on these common complaints? As you leaf through this book, you will see some suggestions and guidelines for prevention and cure which seem rather commonplace. Simply staying out of drafts and taking in plenty of liquids are two examples. But why are these hints helpful? What basic body functions do they serve to normalize, strengthen, and regulate? This booklet answers those questions.

You will notice, however, many unique suggestions, therapies, and insights. The effects of specific attitudes and emotions and a discussion of the acid/alkaline balance within the body are two cases in point. These and other ideas will provide you with a new approach to the cold and flu.

Finally, the key to the valuable information contained in this booklet comes down to one word—application. The Cayce readings invite us not only to consider their perspective, but also to put it to the test. To that end, enjoy this book and follow its suggestions to better health.

Eric Mein, M.D.
Meridian Institute

Chapter 1

OUR BODIES KNOW BEST

THE MIRACLE OF HEALING

You and I are walking miracles, more complex than much of the machinery we are surrounded by in our daily lives. Our nervous systems are more intricate than the computer relays and networks that power and direct the space shuttle *Atlantis*. Our elimination systems are more involved and specific to their tasks than a water purification plant that serves thousands of homes and businesses. If we were called upon to repair and maintain a complex network of computers, most of us would not know where to begin. But our bodies are different. Complex though they are, the power to maintain and heal them is ours.

Science is at a loss to explain where the "wisdom" for the healing process originates. We do not consciously rush Helper T cells to the site of infection. In fact, most of us wouldn't know a Helper T cell if it joined us for dinner! But our bodies not only know these cells, they can scramble them to our defense even before we know we're sick.

THE SPIRIT WITHIN

The Cayce readings are emphatic about the source of this wisdom. Time and time again, the readings revealed that "all *healing* is from the Divine within . . . " (1173-6) And that divinity inspires and directs every cell to perform its unique mission.

Nothing short of miracles results.

Our cells, organs, and tissues perform intricate, life-giving tasks on a daily basis—without our knowledge and without our conscious help. On a given day three to eight billion cells die while an equal number are regenerated. Our blood courses through over 60,000 miles of intricate passageways and arrives on time and without mishap. We are not consciously involved in any of these functions, and yet they happen with precision and purpose.

But, if our bodies are so wise, why do we occasionally become ill?

The bottom line might be hard to swallow. The truth is that we often override our body's innate performance with our own poor judgment. Think, for a moment, of what would happen if you filled your car's gas tank with water. It's easy to imagine the results. Now think of the day last week when you were rushed for time and consumed little more than a fast-food breakfast, skipped lunch, and overate at dinner. Although you did many

2

unwise things, you kept going. That's better than you can say for your car when you failed to provide it with its proper "nourishment."

The difference is that your body's inner wisdom went on overdrive to compensate for lack of appropriate nutrition. It will continue to compensate on your behalf—until it tires of your neglect and sends you a warning in the form of illness.

Perhaps the rushed day I described looks hauntingly familiar. And, perhaps you're down with a cold or flu as you read this book. It's not because your body isn't wise—it's because it's not getting the attention from you it deserves.

Chapter 2

COMMON COLD
OR FLU?

THE UNPLEASANT FACTS

Although past bouts with the common cold and flu tend to blur in our memories, these illnesses are actually separate and distinct viruses. As such, they have different effects on our bodies, resulting in a wide range of unpleasant miseries.

COMMON COLD SYMPTOMS

Runny nose. Watery eyes. Sore throat. Mild temperature. Sneezes. The *gradual* onset of these symptoms usually heralds the arrival of the common cold—a condition where there is acute inflammation of the air passages of the head and throat. Caused by a virus which infects the upper respiratory tract, the common cold leaves the system weakened and symptom-ridden. Our mucous membranes are inflamed, our nose is intermittently stopped up and runny, and we are left literally gasping for air.

We become infected and contagious two to three days prior to the onset of any symptoms and remain contagious throughout the duration of the virus infection. Although the virus can be airborne by a violent sneeze or cough, it is more often transmitted through touch. This contact can be as direct as a handshake or as indirect as a newspaper being passed from a person who is infected to someone who is not. Follow this contact with an innocent rubbing of eye or nose and those germs have landed right where they want to be.

FLU SYMPTOMS

Fever. Chills. Muscular aches and pains. Hacking cough. Hoarseness. When the onset of these symptoms is *sudden*, often overtaking a "well" body in a matter of a few short hours, it is probable that you have come down with the flu. Unlike the common cold, the flu is not localized in the upper respiratory tract, though many of its symptoms are felt there, but is more widespread throughout the body and thus more serious. It is more likely that the flu, if not taken seriously, will leave you vulnerable to bacterial infections, which can lead to bronchitis, pneumonia, ear infections, and the like.

After your body has accepted a flu virus, it takes a relatively short time for the symptoms to appear—usually two days. A person with the flu is highly contagious on the first three days after the symptoms

5

appear, though some people may remain contagious a day or two more. Again, unlike the common cold, transmission of the virus is more often through the air—though it, too, can be transmitted by touch.

ENTER THE IMMUNE SYSTEM

Many medical professionals and lay people alike are in agreement that the immune system will be the focus of much medical and consumer concern in the 1990s—just as cholesterol was in the 1980s. The advent of the AIDS virus challenges researchers to explore new ground—and individuals to take measures to build and maintain an optimum level of immunity.

Simply coming in contact with a virus will not always result in "catching" a cold or flu. If the immune system is strong and the numerous body systems are in balance, a virus can be defeated.

Simply stated, the immune system is the body's internal defense force which seeks out foreign invaders and destroys them. This team is made up of approximately a trillion white blood cells called leucocytes. These cells are found not only in the blood, but also in the lymph and body tissues.

They are your front line of defense.

These white protectors come in many sizes and shapes—from Helper T cells which help identify invaders so that antibodies can be created to phagocytes which literally gobble up foreign microorganisms and cells.

If these cells are strong, healthy, and plentiful, your chances of winning the cold war are in your favor. If they are weak and understaffed, you're a sitting duck to whatever viruses are being passed around the home, office, even shopping mall.

What makes your white blood cells healthy?

The answer is simple. They are directly affected by your body's general health index. If you eat well, exercise regularly, and have a positive outlook on life, your white blood cells will benefit. And so will your attendance record at work.

PIONEERING INSIGHTS INTO THE IMMUNE SYSTEM

In many ways the Cayce readings provided pioneering insights into what strengthens this silent white army. They draw a picture of the body as a complex organism of interdependent body systems. In the case of fighting the common cold, four areas were pinpointed which, if healthy, can help you win the battle. The first three have to do with your physical body. Diet—especially as it affects your acid/alkaline balance, eliminations, and circulation—all play a vital role. Team them up with your emotions, get them all in sync, and you've got a fighting chance against any invader.

Team play *is* the operative strategy. Maintaining the proper acid/alkaline balance while neglecting your circulation will not free you from the threat of a cold. Nor will maintaining a positive attitude while eating an overabundance of acid-forming foods safeguard you against illness.

But there's good news. There are many daily therapeutic regimens you can follow which will help you maintain and restore the balance which is your body's

7

natural condition. Many of these practices are as simple as eating the right foods and getting plenty of rest. Others might require a bit more vigilance—like thinking positive thoughts and forgiving those with whom you have problems! Nevertheless, it is important that you do these and incorporate them into your healing regimen.

Chapter 3

PREVENTION IS POSSIBLE

CHOKE A COLD TO DEATH

Follow these four steps to stay cold- and flu-free during the winter season:

1. Eat right to maintain your acid/alkaline balance
2. Maintain healthy eliminations
3. Stimulate circulation
4. Think positively

This strategy will enhance your body's immune system so that it's ready to fight off even the most persistent cold and flu germs. The Cayce readings were clear on this point. "Precautions in all these directions to keep a near normal balance are measures best to be taken towards preventing the contracting of cold." (902-1) In another reading Cayce added, "But if a body is sufficiently balanced as to make for resistance, there will be sufficient leukocytes in the blood supply to choke a cold to death immediately!" (386-3)

THERE'S NO BETTER TIME
THAN THE PRESENT

I would recommend that you adopt these suggestions as soon as possible.

However, rigorously implementing them during the cold and flu season, either when you're aware a cold is "going around" or when you're actually starting to feel some mild symptoms, might serve to hold your illness at bay and mobilize your body's natural defense system.

YOUR ACID/ALKALINE BALANCE

The Cayce readings indicated that cold and flu germs thrive in an acid system.

The natural acid/alkaline state of our bodies is a pH of 7.4 (i.e., slightly alkaline); below 7 is more acid, above 7 is more alkaline. Although the blood remains constant at 7.4, other body fluids can fluctuate. When asked what precautions could be taken against the common cold, the readings replied, "Keep alkalized." (480-45)

What causes an overacid system? Poor diet, sluggish eliminations, being physically run down, even negative thinking.

HOW TO TEST YOUR ACID/ALKALINE STATE

The best way to test your acid/alkaline balance is by using blue litmus paper (found at most drugstores) to determine the pH of your saliva. The best time to make this test is in the morning before eating or drinking. Take a paper strip and wet it with your saliva. If the paper remains blue in color, the pH is alkaline at 7.0 or above. You're in safe territory.

If the strip turns pink, your saliva pH is below 7.0 or acid. Since you are most susceptible to colds and flu when in an acid state, you need to take immediate measures to restore your acid/alkaline balance, primarily through your diet.

WHAT YOU EAT MATTERS

The Cayce readings indicated that we should keep "about a twenty percent acid-producing to an eighty percent alkaline-producing diet." (949-14) What the readings mean when they refer to the acid- or alkaline-"producing" effects of particular foods is how they react chemically when your body metabolizes them. In general, alkaline-producing foods include fruits and vegetables; acid-producing foods encompass, primarily, meats and cereals.

COLD PREVENTION DIET

Alkaline-Forming Foods
(80% of Your Diet)

All fruits except cranberries, plums, and prunes
All vegetables except for lentils and corn
All milk, including buttermilk
Almonds, brazil nuts, chestnuts, coconut, hazelnuts
Coffee, tea, molasses, brown sugar, brewer's yeast

Acid-Forming Foods
(20% of Your Diet)

All meats except for mincemeat
All cereals and bakery products except for soybeans
All cheeses and eggs
Peanuts, pecans, walnuts

Adhere to the percentages in this diet and you'll feel better than ever.

COMBINING FOR VALUE

In addition to watching your intake of acid- and alkaline-forming foods, Cayce made specific recommendations regarding what foods combine well with others. According to the readings, poorly combining foods can create toxins which impede the immune system. Use the following "Food-Combining Guidelines" to receive the optimum nutritional value and benefits from the foods you eat (by not combining first and third columns):

FOOD-COMBINING GUIDELINES

Food Type	Friendly	Unfriendly
Starches	Vegetables	Milk, fruits, eggs, cheese, nuts, meats, sweets
Meats, seafood, fowl, nuts	Vegetables	Starches, milk, fruits, sweet desserts, cheese

Food Type	Friendly	Unfriendly
Vegetables	All foods	
Dairy	Vegetables, fruits	Starches, meats, fish, fowl
Fruits (sweet)	Vegetables, dairy	Meats, fowl, seafood, eggs
Fruits (tart)	Vegetables	Starches, milk

A FINAL WORD ON VEGETABLES

As you can see, vegetables are highly recommended in the readings. Not only are they alkaline-reacting in nature, they're friendly to all other food types—a condition which translates into being user-friendly for you!

Here are three other tidbits of advice which the readings offered for planning your vegetable menu:

■ Eat locally grown vegetables. They are fresher and healthier for your body.

■ Prepare your vegetables raw or steamed in Patapar paper (available at health food stores).

■ Combine in your salad at least three vegetables from above the ground to every one below the ground.

EAT SLOWLY WITH A THANKFUL ATTITUDE

The Cayce readings indicated that bolting down food is a primary culprit in causing colds. Also, eating while upset or angry can have adverse effects on your health. In many ways, it's not simply *what* you eat that's important, it's *how* you eat as well.

So, slow down and enjoy your meals. Cayce indicated that chewing foods thoroughly not only helps with digestion and assimilation but also helps keep the glands of the neck and face healthy.

And, as you eat, visualize the positive effects a healthy balanced meal will have on your body and your energy level. Combine this with a thankful attitude, and you'll reap health-filled rewards.

CAN VITAMIN SUPPLEMENTS HELP?

Nutrition experts as well as Cayce agree that the optimum source of all vitamins and minerals is from unprocessed, natural foods. In the instances where Cayce did recommend vitamin supplements, he strongly suggested that they be taken only for short periods of time, especially when the body is run down for one reason or another.

The readings did not recommend megadoses of supplements and warned that taking vitamins over an extended period of time can impair the body's ability to extract them from normal food intake. And, there's an added danger. An excess of certain vitamins in the body can be as harmful as a vitamin deficiency.

THERE'S VALUE IN FOODS

In short, there are four vitamins and one mineral that can help you get ready for the cold season. Here's what they do and where you can find them.

Vitamin A promotes healthy mucous membranes, stimulates the thymus gland, which produces Helper T cells, and according to the Cayce readings is important to lymph circulation. Natural sources of this vitamin include liver, carrots, green and yellow vegetables, yellow fruits, eggs, and dairy products.

B Complex strengthens the immune system and is also important to the mucous membranes. Cayce recommended the B vitamins more often than any other vitamin, noting that they cannot be stored by the body and must be taken daily. Natural sources of it include whole grains, brewer's yeast, brown rice, wheatgerm, liver, eggs, cheese, and milk.

Vitamin C is widely considered an important remedy for the common cold. Like the B vitamins, it is not stored by the body. However, it strengthens the immune system and helps fight bacterial infection, thus a daily intake is critical. Natural sources include green leafy vegetables, citrus fruits, berries, tomatoes, cauliflower, and potatoes.

Vitamin E assists white blood cells in resisting infection. Natural sources include wheatgerm, soybeans, vegetable oils, shrimp, green leafy vegetables, whole wheat, and whole grains.

Zinc has stolen the limelight from vitamin C in current research on the immune system. Findings indicate that this mineral increases the production of Helper T cells. Natural sources include lamb, oysters, wheatgerm, brewer's yeast, and eggs.

Luckily, although many of the above food sources overlap, there's still lots of variety as well. Eat plenty of them year round and your white blood cells will be ready for deployment when the "cold alarm" sounds.

GELATIN—A HEALTHY DESSERT AT LAST!

One interesting idea from the readings was the statement that gelatin, acting as an enzyme, aids in the absorbtion of nutrients. A fruit salad prepared with gelatin or the mixing of gelatin with fresh fruit juices are excellent ways to increase the body's intake of vitamins from natural foods.

SUGGESTED VITAMIN REGIMEN

First, I would suggest you heed the Cayce recommendation regarding the intake of gelatin as described above. Make it a part of your daily routine. Also, consider including in your daily diet generous portions of the foods listed on p. 15. Finally, when you are feeling particularly run down or under stress, I recommend a good B-complex vitamin which includes C and zinc. Additionally, a vitamin A supplement might also benefit you. There are several on the market, so consult with your physician or pharmacist to find one that seems right for you.

Take these vitamins for two weeks, then leave off for one week. Continue with this regimen until you feel your energy is restored.

ELIMINATIONS

Another physical condition which leaves us vulnerable and more likely to catch a cold is a sluggish or improperly functioning elimination system. A buildup of wastes and toxins breaks down our immunity and provides an ideal environment for cold germs to multiply.

Although many people tend to think of the kidneys, liver, and colon as being the primary players in insuring proper elimination, we need to remember that the skin and lungs perform an equally vital role.

The Cayce readings stressed that all these parts of the elimination systems should be kept in balance. Focusing on improvement in one area without a plan of action in the others could result in one overactive and overtaxed system, while the other systems remain inert and sluggish.

Where do all these wastes originate? Not surprisingly, from both foreign and domestic sources.

Internally, the day-to-day functioning of our body's cells burns energy and creates byproducts, which the Cayce readings called ash. Additionally, in the normal course of a day, hundreds of billions of our body's cells die as others are regenerated. These wastes must be removed from the body.

Also our food intake from external sources can come replete with dangerous additives and sometimes nutritionally empty calories. Compounding our sometimes deficient dietary intake are environmental pollutants we take in through the lungs and skin.

To help us deal with these wastes here are some hints that will help keep these four elimination systems functioning properly.

KIDNEYS

The readings frequently discussed the role of the kidneys in freeing the body of toxic buildup. At the same time they often discussed the role of the liver which, although it rightfully functions as part of the digestive tract, has a vital and important relationship with the kidneys. In short, these two organs work as a team. On the one hand, the liver performs hundreds of metabolic functions through its processing of the blood. On the other hand, the kidneys filter the body's blood several hundred times each day. The readings indicate that a breakdown in the balance between these two organs can cause them to throw the toxins which they help to eliminate back into our systems.

The most important rule in keeping these organs healthy won't surprise you.

Drink 6-8 glasses of water daily. You've heard this suggestion before in dozens of health books. The Cayce readings make the same suggestion, noting that this practice would benefit the kidneys, liver, and colon. And, of course, water is the agent by which toxins are eliminated through the skin.

Here's a suggested routine which will help you to pace yourself to drink this amount of water daily. Note that Cayce recommended that your first half glass of water in the morning be warm because it will help cleanse a relatively empty colon after the nighttime fast.

When	Glasses
Upon arising (warm)	½
Mid-morning and afternoon	2
Before breakfast, lunch, and dinner	3
After breakfast, lunch, and dinner	3
Total	8½

COLON

As mentioned above, water intake will also benefit your colon. Two other suggestions made by Cayce deal with the intake of roughage as a natural laxative as well as colonic irrigations or enemas.

Cayce strongly recommended the consumption of a raw lunch—either a salad or an assortment of raw vegetables. Complement your salad with a slice of whole grain bread. You'll feel better and have a higher energy level all afternoon.

The next step you can take to improve your colon's health is an occasional internal cleansing with water. Unfortunately, the mere mention of a colonic irrigation or enema often lands on unwilling ears, but look at it this way. We bathe our bodies on a regular basis. Depending upon our daily activities, however, our body comes in contact with a minimal amount of dirt and grime. Part of what we wash away are eliminants from our skin and pores. Just think of the waste materials that move through your colon—morning, noon, and night. Many of these particles cling to the walls of your intestines, slowing the passage of wastes. Your general health and immune system suffer as a result. A colonic or a series of enemas on a regular basis will benefit you greatly.

LUNGS

The lungs function as the elimination system for carbon dioxide—an end product of metabolism. Nothing can benefit the lungs more than fresh air and regular, deep breathing.

Deep-breathing exercises were frequently described in the readings. Later, you will learn a morning exercise that incorporates deep breathing. You'll also benefit if, throughout your day, you occasionally pause and take several deep breaths—exhaling each completely and forcefully. Try this simple breathing exercise some afternoon, when you're sitting at your desk, head heavy, eyelids drooping. You'll be surpirsed at how invigorating it can be.

SKIN

The skin is your body's largest organ. Through the skin and sweat glands much of your body's work of throwing off waste is accomplished.

Hydrotherapy and massage were often recommended by Cayce as a means to improve circulation.

One "at-home" routine is to soak in a tub of hot water at least three times a week. Just prior to your bath, massage your body with peanut oil, paying particular attention to legs and feet. This rubdown will stimulate circulation and leave your body soft and smooth afterwards.

Another suggestion is to get a massage on a weekly basis. If you can find a massage therapist whom you like and trust, you will find it easier to keep your regular appointments. Consistency will be your long-term ally. Precede this therapy with a steam bath, as Cayce suggested, and you'll feel relaxed and renewed.

CIRCULATION

In addition to poor elimination, any imbalance in blood and lymph circulation will contribute to lowering your resistances. Hence, cold feet, drafts, a wet head, and sudden changes in temperature do have an effect on the development of a cold—because they disrupt the even flow of these fluids throughout the circulatory system.

The Cayce readings indicate that the arterial and lymphatic circulations work as a team. The blood delivers nutrients to the cells in even the farthest outposts of your body. The lymph removes the wastes released by those cells after nutrients from the blood are absorbed. In short, the blood brings in the groceries, the lymph takes out the trash.

The major difference between the blood and lymph as part of the circulatory system is that the blood has a well-equipped and -designed pump to deliver it to its destination. The lymph, however, has no pump but relies on several bodily activities to stimulate its movement. There are two ways to help move the lymph which will fit well into your daily "prevention" plan—exercise and massage. Both of these will provide the lymph with much needed stimulation and also aid the heart pump in performing its duties.

EXERCISE FOR LIFE!

The readings recommended exercise in hundreds of instances for just as many individuals. There are several general guidelines which can be gleaned from these readings for exercises which are not overly strenuous but which will have positive, long-lasting results.

As with all exercise programs, begin gradually. Work up to a program that feels right for you. Most important, design a routine that fits comfortably into your daily regimen. Little could be more counterproductive than an exercise program that is rushed and dreaded.

WALKING

One reading made the following claim: " . . . walking is the best of any exercise . . . " (2823-2) For general health maintenance a daily walk of a half hour is a moderate but effective cornerstone in your exercise routine. The readings often recommended that this walk be taken after dinner to aid digestion.

MORNING AND EVENING STRETCHES

Cayce gave another general guideline which you should keep in mind when planning your exercise program. Many times he recommended that one "stretch like a cat." Now, I'm sure Cayce would not recommend that we design our program to suit the comic-strip character Garfield, though many of us may feel like this sassy cat when we think about getting started! Rather, he recommended a consistent, persistent routine, one which focused on upper body stretches in the morning and lower body stretches in the evening.

MORNING WAKE-UP

A good exercise for the morning is to stand straight and tall, and gradually rise up on your tip toes, inhaling slowly and deeply, and gently bring your arms upward over the head. Then, bend forward and bring your fingertips down to touch your toes. Just as your hands near the floor, exhale in a single forceful breath. Repeat this three to ten times—whatever is comfortable for you.

Tightening the leg muscles and employing the diaphragm are particularly effective in moving the lymph, which has slowed down a great deal during your night's rest.

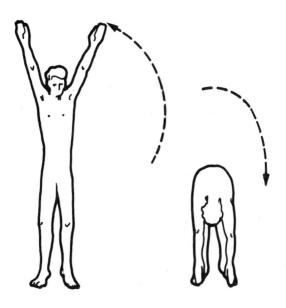

PELVIC ROLL

A specific evening exercise often recommended is the pelvic roll. Position yourself on the floor, face down, as if preparing to do a pushup, but place your feet flush against the wall. Raise yourself up on your arms, then rotate your hips in a circle—three times clockwise, three times counterclockwise. However, if this position is too strenuous, you may actually rest on your elbows rather than your hands when assuming the pushup stance.

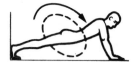 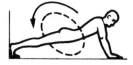

Circular motion

| **clockwise** | **counterclockwise** |
| **three times** | **three times** |

Combine these exercises with other stretching movements for your morning and evening routine.

HEAD AND NECK

Any mention of exercise is not complete without the head and neck roll.

This exercise was recommended in the Cayce readings over three hundred times, making it one of the most frequently recommended routines. It is quite simple and can have particularly positive effects.

Here's how you do it.

Sit with your spine erect and your shoulders relaxed. Bend your head forward three times, backward three times, to the right three times, to the left three times. Then, gently rotate your head 360 degrees in both directions three times. Do this series slowly and deliberately.

This exercise brings more circulation to the head and neck. This increase can help improve sight and hearing.

An added benefit: the increased blood supply in the head and neck area strengthens our body's defense system in the upper respiratory passages and facilitates the lymph's removal of potentially threatening toxins from this body sector.

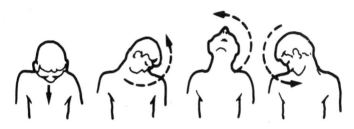

FINAL WORD ON EXERCISE: JUST DO IT!

A popular T-shirt design sports the phrase "JUST DO IT." Dr. Harold J. Reilly, author of *The Edgar Cayce Handbook for Health Through Drugless Therapy,* made a similar point: "The best exercises are the ones you do!" You'll find that once you get into your routine, you'll suffer more from breaking it than from the occasional inconvenience of keeping it up.

MASSAGE

As was mentioned previously, massage can be the master of your fate when it comes to stimulating circulation. Getting these two rivers (blood and lymph) flowing will enable them to do their most important work: to deliver nutrients and dispose of wastes.

Remember, find a massage therapist who provides

the kind of massage you need. Then, set up a standing appointment. Consistency and persistency are the backbones of this particular therapy.

A WORD ON OSTEOPATHY

The Cayce readings often recommended osteopathy for prevention and treatment of a variety of conditions. The cold and flu were no exceptions. An osteopathic or chiropractic adjustment is intended to keep the spine in order, making sure that the signals it sends to various organs via the nervous system are correct. If for any reason the spine is poorly aligned, it may send the wrong signals and may result in an imbalance in any number of body systems.

Occasionally, some individuals were told that the problems in their upper dorsal and cervical spine (or upper back and neck) made them more susceptible, with the least acidity, to catching a cold.

A routine adjustment can benefit circulation and elimination, and thus have an effect on your acid/alkaline balance. Think of it as getting a "body tune-up." You wouldn't neglect your car, so why neglect your body?

ATTITUDES AND EMOTIONS

"Thoughts are things!" This concept permeates the Cayce readings. If you know that a cold is going around and you are fairly certain you're going to catch it, rest assured you will! Not only will this defeatist attitude result in illness, but—according to the readings—feelings of anger and resentment as well are causes for coming down with a cold. One reading suggested a "physio-psycho" remedy: "Instead of snuffing, BLOW! Instead of resentments, LOVE!" (288-44)

Recent research on the psychology of colds has echoed Cayce's insight when it was found that introverts tend to have more colds. Also, those under stress suffer worse cold symptoms than those under less psychological pressure.

Haven't you noticed how your feelings affect your health? Think back to a day when you received some bad news—perhaps your contractor discovered termites in the basement. Your checkbook balance was declining as fast as your blood pressure was rising. You began to feel anxious and uneasy. You even lost your appetite. These feelings had nothing to do with a virus and everything in the world to do with your emotions.

PROOF IS IN THE PLACEBO

You've heard of the placebo effect. You've read about it in magazines. Sugar pills can work to improve a patient's condition—if the patient believes the pills are real. What's at work is the recipient's commitment, *on an emotional level*, to the power of the placebo. The same positive expectancy can help prevent illness—and bring about healing.

POSITIVE EMOTIONS ARE A POSITIVE MOVE TOWARD HEALTH

You may feel that the following suggestions sound much easier than drinking eight glasses of water a day.

Unfortunately for us all, they're not. Maintaining a positive, loving attitude is hard work requiring constant vigilance. In fact, world peace might result if we all heeded this wisdom.

Here are some places to start:

■ Become aware of your feelings. When they're negative, try to understand them. Don't condemn yourself for them, but simply try to discover where they originate.

■ Don't hold resentments. If appropriate, talk your feelings out with the person they involve. You'll usually find that these feelings do concern a relationship of one kind or another. If you can't take this approach, talk them out with God through prayer.

■ Whatever the instance, once you've processed these feelings, forgive. Remember, you may need to forgive another person, or you might need to forgive yourself.

■ Finally, look for the good in bad situations. There's truth in the adage that behind every cloud is a silver lining. If you can believe this, your life will have new meaning—and your body will have a new source of nourishment.

QUICK TIPS TO BEAT THE WINTER BLAHS

You are what you eat. During the cold season, monitor your diet like a hawk. Remember the 20/80 rule of acid/alkaline balance. Don't take any unnecessary risks—like having that evening snack of apple pie. Instead, munch on fresh fruits and raw vegetables, especially carrots and celery. Drink eight glasses of water a day. And don't forget to eat slowly and with a thankful attitude. Consider short-term usage of a vitamin supplement.

Fresh air and exercise. Kill two birds with one stone. Get out for a morning or evening walk and breathe in that fresh air! You'll be stimulating the circulation throughout your body and tossing off toxic wastes as well. Stretch your arms as you go along and even find a quiet spot to sit and rest and reflect on your many blessings.

You learned it in kindergarten. Wash your hands frequently. Those cold germs are most effective if you act as emissary to deliver them directly to your nose or eyes. Keep a stash of fresh tissues on hand and use them frequently.

What you wear counts, too. Tight clothes can restrict circulation. Plus, they tend not to be as warm as a layer or two of nice, soft clothing. Your body thrives on being comfortable. Help it out!

Think positively. You'll feel better all around—and probably have fewer conflicts. And, you'll be surprised at the time you'll save. Think of all the hours spent in working out problems caused by negative thoughts and unkind actions. Now you can use that time for your exercise routine, and everyone will benefit.

Treat yourself to something special. Give yourself a firm, peanut oil rubdown. Then retreat to a nice, hot bath several times a week. Turn on some soothing music and lie back and relax. Afterwards, put on those flannel pajamas, and hop in bed. You'll feel better than you've felt in ages.

Get plenty of rest. A good night's sleep and a quiet moment or two during the day will have a tremendous effect on your health. Get in the habit of retiring early and reading a good book for an hour or so. You'll be relaxed and ready for a good night's sleep—and energized in the morning when you awaken.

Chapter 4

THE THREE R'S OF CURE

CAN THE COMMON COLD BE CURED?

If you've turned directly to this section, chances are you're presently suffering from a cold or flu. Or perhaps you're curious to see if there are any new suggestions here on how to fight one of the oldest and most frequent ailments which plagues humankind. Whatever has led you to this section, you'll find practical and effective advice—some of it old, but much of it new.

As discussed earlier, the common cold and flu are viral infections which are not treatable by antibiotics. Medicines are not a simple panacea for these ailments. The key to curing the common cold and flu lies within your own body.

HOW LONG WILL A COLD LAST?

This is an age-old question. It may be one of curiosity or of dire importance, depending on your current state of health—or illness.

If your immune system is strong and your body is in otherwise good, balanced health, it is possible that you can conquer your cold in as little as 48 hours. However, if you can't boast a strong immune system, the siege will be a bit longer—more likely a week to ten days.

But relief is at hand in the pages that follow. Your symptoms can be made more bearable, with the odds of emerging stronger and healthier being in your favor in the end.

THE THREE R's

Rest, restoration, and *relief* are the three basic R's the Cayce readings stress in curing the common cold. First and foremost, if you're down with a cold, get plenty of rest. Second, restore your body systems to their proper balance. Third, lessen your symptoms with some basic natural remedies that both relieve and restore.

REST

The first "R" stands for rest.

You were in a better position to overcome your cold when you were a child and your mother insisted you stay home from school and rest. More than likely, deep down inside, you knew that she was right. That's why, if you have children, you don't hesitate to keep them home when they're sick. But can you honestly say you do the same for yourself?

One of the greatest threats to health is the unwillingness of many adults to stay at home in bed when they are ill. There's a big meeting we don't want to miss or a deadline we need to meet. There's really no limit to the harm we can cause when we go out in public with a cold. First, we spread it to others. More than likely, that's how you got your cold in the first place. Before it was yours, it was someone else's! Secondly, we subject our already vulnerable body to germs, including the possibility of bacterial infection. Finally, we drain our bodies of the much needed vital energies that are necessary to heal ourselves.

So stay at home, preferably in bed, for at least the first two days. This is the foundation upon which to build your strategy for the cold war.

RESTORE BALANCE

The second "R" represents the need to restore balance.

Once you have committed to resting during your bout with the cold or flu, the readings emphasize the importance of restoring balance within the body systems as the best strategy to "cure" a cold.

Unfortunately, you might need a crystal ball that is tuned in to your body's intricate systems in order to accurately and definitely tell you where the breakdown has occurred. However, a pattern emerges in the readings that suggests a gradual and safe regimen for restoring balance to the vital body systems most likely to be involved in the cold war.

- Your eliminations, acid/alkaline balance, and gastrointestinal tract (stomach and intestines)

- Your circulatory systems

- Your attitudes and emotions

ALKALINIZE/ INCREASE ELIMINATIONS/ REST YOUR GASTROINTESTINAL TRACT

These three tasks all play a vital role in improving your body's internal "environment." The readings stressed that the elimination system serves many purposes, one of which is to flush acids and toxins out of the body. Remember, Cayce indicated that cold and flu germs thrive in an acid environment. Hence the importance of stimulating eliminations to help decrease acidity *while* being sure to take foods that are alkaline-producing. The gastrointestinal tract is processing incoming food and dispatching wastes and—if disturbed—can throw refuse into the upper circulatory system, causing increased irritation and complications to chest, throat, and head. To do its job right, the body requires proper incoming food and a clear channel of eliminations through the alimentary canal.

It is easy to see how vital it is that these systems work in harmony with one another but overwhelming to think of developing a strategy for striking such a balance. Fortunately, the Cayce readings offered several simple suggestions to accomplish this end.

CASTORIA

Castoria not only acts as a laxative to help cleanse the alimentary canal, but also is an effective alkalinizer which aids the liver in processing and eliminating the excess acids in your system. This increased activity of your liver will also help correct circulation imbalance and thus stimulate drainage of facial congestion.

The first day of your cold, while resting in bed, take one sip (¼ teaspoon) of Castoria every hour until you have a full elimination of the alimentary canal. You may find that you will have to sip the entire bottle before this is completely accomplished.

LIQUIDS, LIQUIDS, LIQUIDS

It is also important to consume a light, liquid diet during the first one or two days of your cold, taking in as much water as you can. The Cayce reading on the common cold gave this general instruction: "... the liquid diet is best ... " (902-1) Such a diet will decrease the burden of eliminations and rest the intestinal tract.

CITRUS FRUIT JUICES

Be sure to include as much in the way of citrus fruit juices as you are comfortable with to help alkalinize your system and provide much needed vitamin C. The Cayce readings specifically suggested squeezing the juice of ½ lemon in a large glass of orange juice as an effective cold remedy. Another way to take in citrus fruit juice is by drinking hot lemon water and honey—which will alkalinize the system *and* soothe your aching throat.

SODIUM BICARBONATE

Another route to help alkalinize the system is to drink a glass of water with a teaspoon of sodium bicarbonate added to it. Take this after you awaken in the morning, especially during the first days of your bout with this illness. Another way to consume sodium bicarbonate is to sprinkle a little on a cracker. Or look for "soda" crackers at the store as an easier substitute.

ENEMAS OR COLONICS

When you are feeling mobile, consider obtaining a colonic from a registered health-care provider. Or administer an emema to yourself. Either of these treatments will not only help alkalinize your body but also aid your eliminations. The readings recommended for the colonic a cleansing solution of one teaspoon of salt and one teaspoon of sodium bicarbonate to every gallon

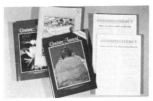

Discover More About

THE EDGAR CAYCE WAY TO HEALTH AND WHOLENESS

BECOME AN A.R.E. MEMBER AND RECEIVE:
★ Membership Magazine   ★ Special Home Studies

YOU ARE ENTITLED TO: ★ Borrow books by mail
★ Names of doctors and health care professionals in your area who use Cayce concepts
★ Edgar Cayce medical readings on loan. Over 300 topics such as:

Arthritis	Headache: Migraine	
Diabetes	Constipation	
Obesity	Emphysema	
Psoriasis	Heart: Angina	
Allergies	Baldness	Moles & Warts
Pyorrhea	Multiple Sclerosis	Scars: Removal
Sinusitis	Cystitis	. . . plus non-medical
Varicose Veins	Indigestion & Gastritis	subjects

FILL IN AND MAIL THIS CARD TODAY:

Enroll me as a member of A.R.E. (Edgar Cayce's *Association for Research and Enlightenment, Inc.*). I enclose $30.00 (Outside U.S.A. add $14.00 postage.)

Method of Payment:
Make check or money order payable to A.R.E.
☐ Check or Money Order   ☐ MasterCard   ☐ VISA
☐ Please bill me later. (U.S.A. only)

Expiration Date

Mo.	Yr.

☐☐☐☐ – ☐☐☐☐ – ☐☐☐☐ – ☐☐☐☐

1280	Signature

Name (please print)

Address

City   State   Zip

📞 **MasterCard or VISA CALL TOLL FREE**
1-800-368-2727 24 hours a day, 7 days a week.

You may cancel at any time and receive a full refund on all unmailed benefits.

785-71

EDGAR CAYCE FOUNDATION and
A.R.E. LIBRARY/CONFERENCE CENTER
Virginia Beach, Va.

OVER 50 YEARS OF SERVICE

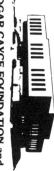

NO POSTAGE
NECESSARY
IF MAILED
IN THE
UNITED STATES

BUSINESS REPLY CARD
First Class Permit No. 2456, Virginia Beach, Va.

POSTAGE WILL BE PAID BY

A.R.E.®
P.O. Box 595
Virginia Beach, VA 23451

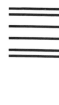

of internal rinse water, followed with a final rinse of one teaspoon of Glyco-Thymoline to one gallon of water.

SPINAL ADJUSTMENT

Many of the readings on the common cold and flu recommended osteopathic treatments to correct possible misalignments of the spine which can hinder elimination of toxins. These readings are very specific to individuals, so you should consult with an expert on spinal mobilizations to determine the best treatment for you.

BALANCE IN CIRCULATION

Once you have taken steps to improve eliminations, to restore your acid/alkaline balance, and to rest your gastrointestinal tract, it's time to pay special attention to another key player in winning the cold war: your blood and lymph circulation. In many ways your circulatory system is the front line in your battle against cold and flu. Both blood and lymph reach your head, throat, and chest, delivering nutrients and virus-fighting cells to the places where they are urgently needed. They also pick up toxins and wastes—the refuse of the war in which germs thrive—and carry them to the proper eliminations depot. Thus, the rationale in the Cayce readings to get the elimination systems in order first, so that they are prepared to deal with the wastes later delivered by the blood and lymph.

What is the best way to stimulate circulation? The answers may seem old-fashioned, but they work.

STAY WARM

Staying warm and dry during your illness will benefit your circulation. Take precautions to keep your feet and hands particularly cozy. They chill easily when you're fatigued, and this condition can disturb the flow of blood and lymph, whose red and white rivers are working hard to provide nourishment to areas that need repair—and remove wastes as well. Join their team by staying warm and dry.

TAKE HOT BATHS

A nice, hot bath will not only make you feel better temporarily, it will also help balance the hepatic circulation. Add two or three tablespoons of mustard to the water for added benefit. Mustard is a known stimulant of circulation. Rub your entire body down afterward with peanut oil or massage your lower back, hips, thighs, and legs with the Mutton Tallow Rub, described in Chapter 5, for extra relief.

ANALYZE ATTITUDES

Working with your mental state is an important step in the restoration process. Throughout the duration of illness and recovery remember Cayce's emphasis on the effects of attitudes and emotions on your body's health index. Specifically he zeroed in on anger and resentment as the ones which create a perfect environment for cold and flu germs to thrive.

You'll more than likely feel vulnerable and depressed

during the worst stages of your illness. You might even resent the timing of your illness—or the person who you feel passed it on to you. Just remember to focus on getting well. As you're doing this, concentrate on the many positive activities you will undertake when you're feeling strong again. The readings stressed that a healthy body should be used to serve others—and not simply to be healthy for health's sake.

In summary, remember these powerful words: "Instead of snuffing, BLOW! Instead of resentments, LOVE!" (288-44)

RELIEF

The final "R" stands for relief.

One of the most important understandings regarding the symptoms you have during a cold or flu is that they are the results of your body's natural defense system in action. For example, a fever is a sign of your body's attempt to fight the virus; a cough loosens congestion so that phlegm can be removed from the lungs.

The readings' approach is unique in that the remedies suggested help relieve symptoms—not eradicate them. What you want is that your symptoms "run their course"—as opposed to being stopped dead in their tracks. Remember that your body has inner wisdom and that "wisdom" deployed your symptoms in the first place.

REMEDIES FOR RELIEF

The following chapter "Remedies for Relief" will benefit you in two ways. First, the remedies described will help relieve your symptoms, allowing you to rest more comfortably. Second, they will aid in the restoration of balance within your body systems.

Chapter Five

REMEDIES FOR RELIEF

WHERE TO FIND THE INGREDIENTS

For ease of reference the remedies are grouped according to your symptoms. You'll immediately notice that many of the ingredients are herbs and substances which you do not have in your medicine chest. But don't be discouraged; you have two options for obtaining these remedies.

First, some are available commercially through your drugstore or health food store. Appendix C has information that will be helpful to you in locating these remedies prepared in advance. Second, the ingredients for the remedies, should you decide to make them in your home, are readily available at most health food stores and some pharmacies.

A GENERAL REMEDY

If you are suffering from a cold which is centralized in your upper respiratory system, this remedy should be the backbone of your treatment. It's the "general" of your army of remedies and is "generally" good for all aspects of your condition.

The key ingredients of this cherry tonic remedy act in the following ways: Ginger is a circulatory stimulant and expectorant. Horehound, too, is a gentle expectorant. Rhubarb complements these two herbs by serving as a mild laxative. The other ingredients act as a base and flavoring for the herbs. In combination, they help decrease cough, maintain expectoration, and increase eliminations. Thus, symptoms are relieved and the body systems are brought back into balance.

Ingredients	Quantity
Distilled water	2 oz.
Honey	2 oz.
Grain alcohol	1 oz.
Syrup of wild cherry bark	1 oz.
Syrup of horehound	½ oz.
Syrup of rhubarb	½ oz.
Elixir of wild ginger	½ oz.

Combine the water and honey and allow the mixture to come to a boil. Then add the grain alcohol. Put in the remaining ingredients in the order given. Take the mixture one teaspoon at a time, as close together as every hour. Always shake the syrup well before each dose.

COUGH AND CHEST CONGESTION

The cold and flu germs have made their way to your lower air passages which respond in the same way as did your nasal airways. Tightness, aching, and congestion in your chest result. Your lungs respond to any foreign substance with their self-cleaning instinct—a cough.

The following three remedies will help break up the congestion so that phlegm can be expelled more easily, allowing the body's cough mechanism to rest.

STEAM INHALANT

The readings recommended a steam inhalant for the relief of lower respiratory congestion. For ease of preparation, here's how to use the same ingredients from the Alcohol Inhalant (described later on p. 45) for another remedy—except for the alcohol.

Ingredients	Quantity
Oil of eucalyptus	20 drops
Compound tincture of benzoin	15 drops
Oil of turpentine	5 drops

Add these ingredients to a pint of boiling water and inhale the steam from nearby—but do not put your face directly over the pan. Or place the mixture in a vaporizer near your bedside.

MUTTON TALLOW RUB

A rub of equal parts of mutton tallow, turpentine, and camphor was frequently recommended in the readings as an upper chest decongestant.

Ingredients	Quantity
Mutton tallow	2 oz.
Turpentine	2 oz.
Camphor	2 oz.

Melt the mutton tallow. Then allow it to cool. Before it congeals add the turpentine and camphor, pouring them down the inside wall of the pan to avoid spattering. Stir them together and store the mixture in a brown container.

Rub it on the upper chest and neck around the glands. In the evening, wrap two thicknesses of cotton flannel around the neck to increase effectiveness. Also, consider applying a heating pad over the flannel to help your body absorb the healing compound.

Label and date the container. Keep up to a year.

ONION POULTICES

Take a large, fresh onion and grind it to a moist pulp. Place the pulp in a small pillow case or cheesecloth bag. Make the poultice ¼-½-inch thick. Apply the pack where you feel the heaviness in your chest. Use in the morning for two to three hours, as you rest in bed. Bathe afterwards. Apply again in the evening. Cayce indicated that this poultice would help reduce inflammation.

NASAL CONGESTION

In defending itself against the invading armies of the virus germs, the body rushes blood to the site to ward off infection. The result is swelling. Coupled with the pressure this creates, the mucous membranes step up the production of mucus to wash away millions of dead and dying cells—the casualties of the cold war. The three remedies mentioned below will help clean your nasal passages, leaving them moist and soothed.

ALCOHOL INHALANT

The Cayce readings gave several formulas for inhalants. Generally, the most common recommendations for the upper respiratory tract included inhalants that contained alcohol. The following inhalant will also help clear chest congestion.

Ingredients	Quantity
Grain alcohol	4 oz.
Oil of eucalyptus	20 drops
Compound tincture of benzoin	15 drops
Oil of turpentine	5 drops

Take an 8-oz. dark glass bottle with a wide mouth. Prepare two holes in the lid. The holes should be large enough to snugly accommodate a plastic straw in each one. Find two rubber stoppers that fit these holes. The stoppers are to be used for storage purposes. I suggest a large vitamin bottle as a resource. Rubber stoppers can generally be found at a hardware store.

Combine the ingredients listed above in the order given.

The solution should fill the bottle to roughly one-half full.

Insert the rubber stoppers in the lid and shake vigorously. Then, uncork both holes and insert the plastic straws so that their ends are *well above* the level of the liquid formula. Then, inhale two to three times through each nostril and alternately through the mouth as well. DO NOT INHALE THE LIQUID FORMULA—only the fumes released from shaking. Repeat two to three times daily.

Label the bottle with the ingredients and date it. Keep for a year. Heavy use will weaken the solution, so you might need to replace it more often.

GLYCO-THYMOLINE SPRAY

Several readings suggested the use of Glyco-Thymoline as a nasal spray. Simply take an empty, sterilized nasal spray container and fill it with Glyco-Thymoline. Use it as needed to help break up nasal congestion.

An added benefit is that Glyco-Thymoline also has an antiseptic effect on cold germs which infect the mucous membranes lining your nasal passages.

GLYCO-THYMOLINE PACK

A Glyco-Thymoline pack can also help relieve nasal congestion and is especially good for sinus problems.

Bring a pan of water to a boil, then remove it from the heat. Place a cloth in the bottom of the pan and set the bottle of Glyco-Thymoline in the water on top of the cloth. Allow it to heat for three to four minutes.

Then, take a cotton cloth which is roughly six inches square and fold it down to three thicknesses. Place it in a cup and pour the warmed solution over it. Wring it out, lie down, and place the pack directly over the nose and sinus area for 15-20 minutes.

HOARSENESS AND COUGH

You'll know when the enemy has attacked your larynx. The result will be a froggy voice—or sometimes worse. Your body is pumping blood to this vocal organ, but it becomes non-vocal in response. The primary purpose of the remedy described below is to soothe the throat. It will also break up chest congestion and thus eliminate the need for strenuous coughing.

LEMON COUGH SYRUP

The following cough syrup is a bit easier to prepare than the other remedies and was given several times in the readings. It was suggested for hoarseness and coughing.

> 1 egg white
> Juice of 1 lemon
> 1 teaspoon of honey
> 2 drops of glycerine

Thoroughly beat the egg white. Add lemon juice slowly, one drop at a time. Add the honey drop by drop, followed by the glycerine.

Take one teaspoon every two to three hours, not to exceed four teaspoons per day. You'll need to prepare this mixture daily.

SORE THROAT

As the war wages, the throat suffers from viral invasion and post-nasal drip. It's also likely that you're breathing through your mouth, thus drying out the mucous membranes in your throat—leaving these sensitive tissues dry and susceptible to viral threat.

The remedy below will act as an antiseptic to kill germs on contact, plus it's soothing as well.

GLYCO-THYMOLINE/LISTERINE GARGLE

Glyco-Thymoline is a mouthwash antiseptic which has an alkalizing effect on the body. Listerine, with which you are probably more familiar, has an acid-forming effect. Cayce suggested gargling with these two mouthwashes alternately, to help balance the body's acid/alkaline state.

The antiseptic nature of both these mouthwashes will help kill cold germs on contact.

FEVER

Fever is your body's attempt to create an environment too hot for cold and flu germs. A mild temperature may make you uncomfortable, but actually might shorten the duration of your illness. However, if your fever reaches 101°, take measures to reduce it. If it will not go down or soars above 102°, see your doctor immediately.

FOOT BATHS

The readings suggested hot foot baths with mustard followed by a rubdown from the knees or hips using the Mutton Tallow Rub (see p. 44).

Find a large bucket or tub and fill it with hot water. Add one or two tablespoons of mustard to the water and stir. Soak your feet for 10-20 minutes, adding hot water when it gets cooler. Then, do your rubdown and you'll be set.

Repeat this foot bath three to four times daily (followed by a rubdown) at least every four hours.

Chapter Six

WINNING THE SEVEN-DAY COLD WAR

Although not all colds are destined to last seven days, some will—especially if you were caught off guard. But whether your cold lasts a few days or several, the following strategy should deliver you stronger and healthier in the end:

DAY 1 *Tuck yourself in.* There is no question as to whether or not you should rest in bed. Not only will you be less likely to encounter other germs, you will be giving your body an opportunity to rally its defenses. Consume only liquids—preferably fruit and vegetable juices, herbal teas, and perhaps some chicken broth. Follow the instructions for sipping Castoria until your alimentary canal is cleansed. This is the first vital step to getting back on track.

DAY 2 *Symptom relief.* If you can, remain in bed, especially if you have a mild temperature. If your symptoms worsen, as they may do on the second day, consult "Remedies for Relief" to determine a plan of action. Once again, consume only liquids, though a bowl of chicken broth and whole wheat crackers might just be in order. Finish the day off with a cup of hot lemon water and honey.

DAY 3 *Slowly but surely.* Today's the day to get up out of bed and begin building strength. Continue working with the remedies you're finding helpful—but add a bit more substance to your diet. Hot cereal for breakfast, a fresh salad for lunch, some broiled fish for dinner. Complement your noon and evening meals with vegetables rich in B vitamins. Take a hot, relaxing bath and go to bed early.

DAY 4 *Over-the-hump day.* Today's the day to think about bundling up and venturing out for some fresh air. Maybe your destination is your osteopath or chiropractor. Tell him or her about your cold—and the way you've treated it. Your doctor might also offer you more advice—and can give you an adjustment with your condition in mind. Stay on your "Cold Prevention Diet" (see p. 11) and tell yourself how good you're beginning to feel. A positive attitude is powerful medicine.

DAY 5 *Back in the saddle.* You can feel comfortable resuming your schedule today, though you must watch for signs of weakness and exhaustion. Don't push your luck. Watch your diet. Take an afternoon nap if possible, and at the very least go to bed early.

DAY 6 *Be thankful for your health.* Consider doing something helpful for someone else today. Maybe a nice gesture for an individual who nursed you through the cold days. Eat well and keep a steady pace. If you tire out a bit, consider drinking a large glass of water followed by the head and neck exercises as a pick-me-up.

DAY 7 *Remember where you've been.* And don't visit again. You're probably feeling better now. Well enough, in fact, to make a big mistake. Don't go outside without wearing something on your head. Skip the heavy meal your appetite began calling for a few days ago. Review Chapter Three, "Prevention Is Possible." It's now more important than ever. Think of this day as the first day of a new, healthy life.

CONCLUSION

Use your illness to create health.

A cornerstone of the Cayce readings' philosophy is to convert your stumbling blocks into stepping-stones. Nowhere does this adage have more application than in the area of health. For instance, it's likely that you may not have read this book unless you were suffering from a cold—an obvious stumbling block. However, we hope that in reading this book you have been given new insights into how your body works. These new ideas will be of tremendous benefit to your body during the cold seasons ahead.

To truly benefit from your stepping-stones, however, you need to apply consistently and persistently the lessons you have learned. If you follow the advice in this book only until you feel better, then lapse into your old habits and patterns, you're more than likely to catch the next cold that goes around.

Become consciously aware of the major body processes you've learned about—diet, eliminations, and circulation—and take loving steps each day to provide your body with the necessary nutrients, activities, and conditions to keep these systems balanced and properly functioning. Always hold a positive attitude and, when negative emotions arise (for they surely will at times in all of us), express them in a positive, helpful way.

Your health will benefit, and so will your life!

APPENDIX A

WHO WAS EDGAR CAYCE?

Edgar Cayce exhibited unusual psychic ability at an early age and soon became known for his remarkable clairvoyant gifts. In a self-induced state, he was able to diagnose illnesses and prescribe remedies with remarkable success. Often referred to as "the sleeping prophet" and the world's most documented psychic, Edgar Cacye left behind a legacy of over 14,000 psychic readings covering such subjects as healing, dreams, meditation, reincarnation, prophecy, and psychic ability.

Born in 1877 in Hopkinsville, Kentucky, he discovered by accident that he could absorb information on any particular subject merely by napping for a while on a book pertaining to that topic. At the age of fifteen he suffered an accident, and, while in a coma, instructed his astonished parents to prepare a poultice to be applied at the base of his brain. The application fully restored him.

After he reached adulthood, his job as a salesman was threatened by a mysterious paralysis of the throat muscles which medical doctors were unable to treat. He consulted a hypnotist, and it was under the subsequent trance that Edgar correctly diagnosed his condition and prescribed an almost immediate cure.

Not long after, Edgar discovered that his gift could be used to help others, and what followed was over forty years of helping people from his self-induced state of unconsciousness. For 22 of these years, his readings were largely confined to medical problems; however, the scope of Edgar's abilities expanded in later years to include such subjects as meditation, dreams, reincarnation, and the Bible.

Edgar Cayce is regarded today as one of the most significant explorers of the human psyche in the twentieth century.

APPENDIX B

HOW THE A.R.E. CAN HELP YOU

A wealth of information from the Edgar Cayce readings is available to you on hundreds of topics, from astrology and arthritis to universal laws and world affairs, through the organization which Edgar Cayce founded in 1931, the Association for Research and Enlightenment, Inc.

The facilities and benefits offered by the A.R.E. include the largest body of documented psychic information anywhere in the world: the 14,263 Cayce readings, copies of which are housed in the A.R.E. Library/Conference Center in Virginia Beach, Virginia. These readings have been indexed under 10,000 different topics and are currently being placed on computer. They are available to the public.

Membership in the A.R.E. is inexpensive and includes benefits such as: the bimonthly magazine, *Venture Inward;* home-study lessons in spiritual awareness and growth; the A.R.E. Library, available to you through book-borrowing by mail, offering collections of the actual Edgar Cayce readings as well as access to one of the world's best parapsychological book collections; and the names of doctors or health care professionals in your area who are willing to work with the remedies prescribed in the Edgar Cayce readings.

As an organization on the leading edge of exciting new fields of study, A.R.E. also presents seminars around the nation, led by prominent authorities in various fields and exploring such areas as parapsychology, dreams, meditation, personal growth, world religions, reincarnation and life after death, and holistic health.

The unique path to personal growth outlined in the Cayce readings is developed through a worldwide program of study groups. These informal groups meet weekly in private homes—right in your community—for friendly consciousness-expanding discussions.

A.R.E. maintains a visitors' center that offers a well-stocked bookstore, exhibits, classes, a movie, and audiovisual presentations to introduce seekers from all walks of life to the fascinating concepts found in the Cayce readings.

A.R.E. conducts ongoing research into the helpfulness of both the medical and nonmedical readings, often giving members the opportunity to participate in the studies themselves.

For more information and a free color brochure, write or phone:

A.R.E., P.O. Box 595
67th Street and Atlantic Avenue
Virginia Beach, VA 23451, (804) 428-3588

APPENDIX C

WHERE TO FIND THE
REMEDIES AND INGREDIENTS

Some of the formulations mentioned in the Edgar Cayce readings are available from:

Home Health Products
P.O. Box 3130
Virginia Beach, VA 23454

APPENDIX D

EDGAR CAYCE READING
ON THE COMMON COLD

902-1   2/17/41

Mrs. Cayce: You will have before you the human ailment known as the common cold. You will give information, advice and guidance as to how people may so conduct themselves as to avoid the common cold, or—having contracted a cold—to cure it. You will then answer the questions, as I ask them.

Mr. Cayce: Yes.

As we find, much has been written in many places respecting such, and much has been given through these channels respecting the various stages and the cure—or helpful applications.

For, it is a universal consciousness to the human body. Thus it is almost as individual as all who may contract or even come in contact with such.

Each body, as so oft considered, is a law unto itself. Thus what would be beneficial in one for prevention might be harmful to another; just as what might have beneficial effects upon one might prove as naught to another.

The cold is both contagious and infectious. It is a germ that attacks the mucous membranes of nasal passages or throat. Often it is preceded by the feeling of flushiness or cold sensations, and by spasmodic reactions in the mucous membranes of the nasal passages.

Then, precautionary or preventative measures respecting the common cold would depend upon how this may be fully judged in the human body, or as to what precautionary measures have been taken and as to what conditions exist already in the individual body.

First: A body is more susceptible to cold with an excess of acidity *or* alkalinity, but *more* susceptible in case of excess acidity. For, an alkalizing effect is destructive to the cold germ.

When there has been at any time an extra depletion of the vital energies of the body, it produces the tendency for an excess acidity—and it may be throughout any portion of the body.

At such periods, if a body comes in contact with one sneezing or suffering with cold, it is more easily contracted.

Thus precautions are to be taken at such periods especially.

To be sure, this leaves many questions that might be asked:

Does draft cause a cold? Does unusual change in dress? Does change in temperature? Does getting the clothes or the feet damp? etc.

All of these, to be sure, *affect* the *circulation;* by the depletion of the body-balance, the body-temperature or body-equilibrium. Then at such times if the body is tired, worn, overacid or overalkaline, it is more susceptible to cold—even by the very changes produced through the sudden unbalancing of circulation, as from a warm room overheated. Naturally when overheated there is less oxygen, which weakens the circulation in the life-giving forces that are destructive to *any* germ or contagion or such.

Then if there is that activity in which the body becomes more conscious of such conditions, this of itself *uses* energies oft that produces *psychologically* a susceptibility!

Consequently, as we find, this is one of the most erratic conditions that may be considered as an ill to the human body.

Much at times may also depend upon the body becoming immune to sudden changes by the use of clothing to equalize the pressures over the body. One that is oft in the open and dresses according to the general conditions, or the temperatures, will be *less* susceptible than one who often wraps up or bundles up too much— *unless—unless* there are other physical defects, or such conditions in the system as to have reduced the vitality locally or as a general condition through the system.

So much, then, as to the susceptibility of an individual or body to colds.

Then, precautions should be taken when it is known that such tendencies exist; that is, weakness, tiredness, exhaustion, or conditions arising from accidents as of draft, dampness of clothes, wet feet or the like, or contact with those suffering with a cold.

As is known, all vital forces are activities of the

glandular system; and these are stimulated by specific glandular activity attributed to the functioning of certain portions of the system.

Then, when exposed to such—under the conditions as indicated, or the many other phases of such that make up the experience of an individual, these would be the preventative measures:

The use of an *abundant* supply of vitamins is beneficial, of *all* characters; A, B, B-1, D, E, G and K.

Vitamins are not as easily overcrowded in the system as most other boosters for a general activity. For, these are those elements that may be *stored*—as it were—in their proper relationships one to another, to be called into use when needed or necessary.

This does not mean that it may not be overdone as a preventative, or in cases where infection already exists. For, that which may be helpful may also be harmful—if misapplied—whether by the conscious activity in a body or by an unconscious activity in the assimilating forces of a system. If this were not true, there would never be an unbalancing of *any* portion of the functioning system; neither would there be the lack of coordination or cooperation with the various organs in their attempt to work together.

It is true that the functioning system (assimilating, distributing and eliminating system) attempts to create that necessary for a balance. Yet it can only use that it has at hand. Thus, with a deficiency of any structural building, blood building or tissue building influence, it may cause weakness by drawing on that necessary to supply the needed conditions for the system's balance.

For instance, if there is a bone fracture the body of

itself creates that element to knit this fracture or broken area. Yet it does not supply or build as much of such element during the periods when the fracture does not exist. Hence when it exists, unless there is an abundant supply of that needed—by or from that assimilated—other portions of the body will suffer.

Know that the body must function as a unit. For, one may get one's feet wet and yet have cold in the head! One may get the head wet and still have cold in the head! The same is true in any such relationships. For, the circulation carries the body forces in same, in the corpuscles, the elements or vitamins needed for assimilation in every organ. For, each organ has within itself that ability to take from that assimilated that necessary to build itself. One wouldn't want a kidney built in a lung; neither would one want a heart even in the head (yet it is necessary to function mentally that way often!).

These are conditions to be considered in preventing as well as in correcting colds. Hence it may be said that the adding of vitamins to the system is a precautionary measure—at all seasons when the body is the most adaptable or susceptible to the contraction of cold, either by contact or by exposure or from unsettled conditions.

The diet also should be considered—in that there is not an excess of acids or sweets, or even an excess of alkalinity, that may produce such a drawing upon some portion of the system (in attempting to prepare the assimilating system for such activity in the body) as to weaken any organ or any activity or any functioning as to produce greater susceptibility.

Hence there should be kept a normal, well balanced diet that has proven to be right for the individual body—if precautionary measures are to be taken through such periods.

Also there should be precautions as to the proper clothing, as to drafts, as to dampness of feet, as to being in too hot or too cold a room, as to getting too tired or exhausted in any way or manner.

Precautions in all these directions to keep a near normal balance are measures best to be taken towards preventing the contracting of cold.

When once the cold has attacked the body, there are certain measures that should always be taken.

First, as has so often been indicated, *rest!* Do not attempt to go on, but *rest!* For, there is the indication of an exhaustion somewhere, else the body would not have been susceptible. Then, too, the inflammation of the mucous membranes tends to weaken the body, so that there is the greater susceptibility to the weakened portions of the body throughout the special influence of the lymph and emunctory activity—such as the head, throat, lungs, intestinal system. Then, if there has been an injury in any structural portions of the body, causing a weakness in those directions, there becomes the susceptibility there for the harmful effects from such.

Then, find or determine next where the weakness lies. Is it from lack of eliminations (which causes many ailments)?

Hence quantities of water, as well as an alkalizer, as well as a booster to assimilating forces, are beneficial things towards producing a balance so that the cold and its consequences may be the more readily or easily eliminated or eradicated.

Do not neglect to take the precautions first. Then if

there is the contraction, determine the weakened factor; knowing that what will aid that portion of the body to more easily attain an equilibrium will prove to be the most beneficial.

Many things in many ways are beneficial to those who have contracted cold—dependent, to be sure, upon the general constitution of the body, the amount of vitamins stored in the system, and so on. Also the response depends greatly on whether or not there is the opportunity given for rest, and the not eating too much, so that the body may be aroused to gain its equilibrium.

Hence it is necessary that there be given the booster for those portions of the body needing the stimulation; and those elements that produce more of vital energies are the more helpful influences.

Ready for questions.

Q-1. *What diet is recommended once the cold has been contracted?*

A-1. This depends upon what is the condition. It may be one cause or another that has weakened the system. More generally, the liquid diet is best—or that the more easily assimilated that carries the greater strengthening ability to all portions of the body. Not heavy or solid foods then. Little of meats, unless given at the period of recuperation when those the more easily assimilated would be the better—such as fish, fowl or lamb—never fried, however.

Q-2. *Is the absence of meat in the diet an important factor in avoiding colds?*

A-2. Not necessarily. It depends upon the combinations, rather than any one element that may be singled out as producing destructive forces. If rare meats are taken, or those that have the life in same, in such measures as to set up a weakening of some portion of the digestive forces, in the attempt of the body to assimilate, it may produce a condition of susceptibility. In that case meat should be avoided by that particular body, or in such quantities at least.

Q-3. Do ultraviolet ray lamps help to prevent colds?

A-3. There are periods when the ultraviolet ray may be a factor in preventing such. The body is less susceptible to colds in the summer periods, when there is more of the violet ray obtained from the activity of the sun and its radiations or radionic activity upon the body. Hence in the winter periods when there is the lack of sunshine, or when there is little of it absorbed by the body, the use of such rays at times would naturally be beneficial; though it may be *overdone.*

Q-4. Are osteopathic treatments of particular value in the case of a cold?

A-4. It depends upon what they are for, and at what stage given. If there is tautness by draft upon portions of the body, either from exposure at time of sleeping or at time of general activity, the relaxing of the body through osteopathic treatments is *most* beneficial as a preventative measure. Let this be considered in relationship to osteopathy:

As a *system* of treating human ills, osteopathy—*we* would give—is more beneficial than most measures that may be given. Why? In any preventative or curative measure, that condition to be produced is to assist the system to gain its normal equilibrium. It is known that each organ receives impulses from other portions of the system by the suggestive forces (sympathetic nervous system) and by circulatory forces (the cerebrospinal system and the blood supply itself). These course through the system in very close parallel activity in *every* single portion of the body.

Hence stimulating ganglia from which impulses arise—either sympathetically or functionally—must then be helpful in the body gaining an equilibrium.

Q-5. At what stage in the development of a cold should an individual be isolated from others so as to prevent spread of a cold?

A-5. At the time the temperature produces an unbalancing, or when there is sneezing or coughing. For, these are as precautionary measures of the system in attempting to throw off the germ itself. It is much the same as a horse wagging its tail to eradicate a fly that bites it! If there is pressure upon the mucous membranes, there is the convulsion or spasmodic reaction to eradicate or to throw off the germ that is biting in, see? This then is thrown off by cough or sneeze and is contagious and infectious by mere contact, see?

Q-6. In a general way, any medicines or remedies recommended?

A-6. As has been indicated.

We are through for the present.